Legal & Disclaimer

The information contained in this book and its contents is not designed to replace
or take the place of any form of medical or professional advice; and is not meant to
replace the need for independent medical, financial, legal or other professional
advice or services, as may be required. The content and information in this book
has been provided for educational and entertainment purposes only.

The content and information contained in this book has been compiled from
sources deemed reliable, and it is accurate to the best of the Author's knowledge,
information and belief. However, the Author cannot guarantee its accuracy and
validity and cannot be held liable for any errors and/or omissions. Further, changes
are periodically made to this book as and when needed. Where appropriate and/or
necessary, you must consult a professional (including but not limited to your
doctor, attorney, financial advisor or such other professional advisor) before using
any of the suggested remedies, techniques, or information in this book.

Upon using the contents and information contained in this book, you agree to hold
harmless the Author from and against any damages, costs, and expenses, including
any legal fees potentially resulting from the application of any of the information
provided by this book. This disclaimer applies to any loss, damages or injury
caused by the use and application, whether directly or indirectly, of any advice or
information presented, whether for breach of contract, tort, negligence, personal
injury, criminal intent, or under any other cause of action.

You agree to accept all risks of using the information presented inside this book.

You agree that by continuing to read this book, where appropriate and/or
necessary, you shall consult a professional (including but not limited to your
doctor, attorney, or financial advisor or such other advisor as needed) before using
any of the suggested remedies, techniques, or information in this book.

ACKNOWLEDGEMENTS

*H*ealth is the most blessed and wonderful gift anyone could ever ask for. And the second greatest gift is the unconditional love and care from my wonderful family who has never given up on me with all the struggles that I have been facing since young. To me, obesity has always been a big fear of an obstacle to overcome. Naming of a few illnesses I've had since young, such as acute and high blood pressure, which really makes me feels like a patient and having to be cautious of what I'm eating and not being able to do what I love as well as hanging out as often as I do in the past with my friends based on my current circumstances.

I hereby would like to express my gratitude to my parents for not giving up on me and always being there spot on by my side, going through every single obstacle together with me. Feeling as though they were in the same situation as I was which made me felt guilty as their only son. But nevertheless, it's all over and I would love to share my knowledge and experience that I have gained through changing my life with this guide I created.

Lastly, but most importantly, I want to say a big "**THANK YOU**" to all my readers – yes, that's you! – For giving me an opportunity to help impact and change lives. Your support is very much appreciated; I am both humbled and honoured to be serving you the best I could.

INTRODUCTION

*M*odern lifestyle has led to a large section of the population becoming obese or overweight. While the primary culprit blamed for the issue is a sedentary lifestyle, extensive research suggests that our dietary choices may be more influential. In this book, we shall present various recipes with about 5 ingredients and simple cooking procedures that will significantly assist your weight loss efforts by supplying your body with the appropriate nutrients and maintaining your metabolism.

But before we do that, it is necessary to build a comprehensive understanding of the idea of weight loss, and how our recipes and diet suggestions work. If you have a proper understanding of the science behind it, it is more likely that you will take an approach which will consider all aspects of health and weight loss. Such an approach which includes both moderate exercise as well as proper diet, with our suggested recipes, will help you take a pursue a highly effective strategy for losing weight. After all, there is no point in making progress in one aspect and regressing in others. It will be like taking one step forwards and two steps backward, and you will be going nowhere.

HOW I STUMBLED UPON METABOLISM MIRACLE DIET

*A*fter going through all the hardships with my family, suffering from such severe illnesses since young, waking up in the middle of the night feeling as though someone was holding my heart and squeezing it. The pain continued for hours, I'm unable to call out to my parents for help. All I could do is to curl myself up, hugging my legs as tight as possible and enduring the pain till it slowly fades away... My life felt so miserable, and as I was about to give up... I ended up giving myself two choices. One, start doing something I've never done before and change my life forever, to become even better and healthier, not wanting my parents to worry about me. Two, continue suffering from all the late-night pains and misery which only me myself could really understand how it felt and how big the burden is to my parents...

So, I started looking for a diet that could help reduce my weight (my goal was to lose that excess 70 pounds) while reducing the risk of my illnesses and helps to regain my health at the same time.

I came across a recommendation from a friend, and that's where I stumbled upon Metabolism Miracle Diet. Having the "do or die" mind-set, I decided to take the "trial and error" approach by placing my health on the line to become my own "lab rat".

HOW MY LIFE TOOK A COMPLETE 180-DEGREE TURN

On-going for 2 weeks, the results were in:

1. My high blood pressure dropped from a risky 160/100 down to a healthy range of 110/80.
2. I lost 18 pounds.

I am TRULY excited with the results achieved as this has never happened to me before. I have returned to a much healthier state and being able to consume the foods I love as well! A month later, I have lost more than 40 pounds... and counting.

From then on, I've been sharing my personal experience and knowledge with my family, friends, and relatives. To my surprise, my aunt whom we've never been in contact for years contacted me. Telling me about how big of an idol I was to her after seeing such a huge difference in her transformation.

Thus, regaining her health and cutting down excess pounds on her body that has been creating unnecessary illnesses for her as well as lymphedema which has been bothering her for years. Since then, I've started writing books to share my knowledge with the rest of the world, and that's how this book was created.

THE PROBLEM WITH OBESITY

With the advancements in the treatment of the various pathogenic diseases which used to be the leading cause of deaths for most of human history, today many other kinds of diseases are the leading of poor health and death. Obesity and being overweight is linked to or is a cause of a significant number of such diseases. Cardiovascular problems, such as heart attack and stroke, are very strongly linked to obesity. Obesity can also significantly increase of certain kinds of cancer. Also, millions of people live with chronic conditions such as diabetes which is caused by obesity. Such health issues can be very difficult and expensive to manage. It is much more effective and efficient if you manage your health to avoid getting obese. As the saying goes, 'Prevention is better than cure'.

Understanding Bodyweight

In your quest to attain great health and lose any extra weight, it is highly beneficial to take a moment to understand the weight distribution of the human body. It helps to put things into perspective before we get to the actual weight loss advice.

The composition of body mass would obviously vary from person to person, but for an average healthy adult, muscles make up most of the weight of the body. As you would know already, men have more muscle mass than women, with men having about 45% of their body mass as muscle while women have about 37%. Organs make up about 25% of all the weight in both men and women. Bones make about 15% body mass in men and about 10% in women.

At last, we will be talking about fats, which will be the focus of this book. In healthy adults, fats make up 15% of the body mass in men and about 28% in women. But this percentage can have the largest variability of all the components of body mass. Fat tissue can contribute as little as 5% in very lean adult males to up to 70% of the total body mass in extremely obese individuals. The fat tissue itself is composed of 86% triglyceride and the remaining 14% is mostly water, carbohydrates, proteins and minerals.

You may come to think of fats as an evil or a villainous substance, but it is not. Fats are essential for various bodily functions. In fact, about 5% and 12% of the body mass of men and women respectively are essential fats, which are highly critical for the functioning of bone joints and many other organs. The body creates fats, even if you don't eat them via your food, for a good reason. Besides, fats can be a great source of energy for the body, and they can be stored if necessary.

But as with anything else, too much of anything creates adverse consequences. When the body has too much fat, it causes obesity, leading to various health complications as we had mentioned earlier.

Losing Weight –Exercise vs. Diet Change

When it comes to weight loss, the most important aspect to consider s net calorific intake.

Net calorific intake = calories in – calories out

You must control and reduce your net calorific intake. Whether you educe 100 calories intake or increase physical activity to burn off extra 100 alories, the effect of weight loss will be the same.

While finding various ways to lose weight, it is likely that you will ome across the two major approaches to weight loss. One approach is dding physical activity, preferably some kind of an exercise or regular ports activities. Another involves adapting one's diet to better lose weight. While both aspects are extremely important, the magnitude of the effect of ach of these is not commonly understood by most people.

Let's take an example of an hour cycling as an exercise. One may onsider that committing to dedicate an hour of every day to cycling xercise is a significant commitment. Considering that you do not go on a eisurely bike ride and do it with the intention of exercising, or use a tationary bike in the gym, you are likely to burn about 500 calories. How nuch are 500 calories? You can get 500 calories from a single plain cream agel, or about 4-5 strips of bacon. That's it. You may spend an hour urning those 500 calories or just choose not to eat that one bagel. Clearly, ontrolling diet may be a better option for most people for reducing their et calorific intake.

That does not mean that exercise is not helpful for a healthy lifestyle In fact, exercise is incredibly helpful, its effects on improving one's health are matched by few other changes such as quitting smoking habit. But the amount of exercise required is greatly overestimated by most people. Also most people overestimate the effectiveness of taking up exercise for losing weight. Add to it the commercial interest of food industries to ensure that people keep buying and eating more food, and you have a murky public perception of the benefits of diet change as opposed to exercising.

A moderate intensity exercise for about 30 minutes a day, 5 days a week is enough to achieve most of the benefits of exercise or active lifestyle Such an exercise may be walking briskly; leisurely bicycle rides or even just doing household chores. No extreme physical activity is necessary nor will do any miracles for weight loss.

Keeping Your Metabolism in High Gear

Metabolism is the rate at which your body consumes and uses up nergy. Naturally, you would want your metabolism to be high and ndisturbed to make sure that your body is burning enough calories. We hall discuss a diet plan as well as various recipe in this book to ensure a ood metabolic rate, but there are other factors as well that must be onsidered to ensure good metabolic rate.

Do not adopt extremely low calorie or near starvation diet for losing weight. The body adapts its metabolic functions to how much food it expects to get. f you adopt a near starvation diet, the body considers that you may be carce on food, and thus respond by slowing down your metabolism. This vill significantly reduce the rate at which your body consumes calories, hus significantly reducing of any effort to lose weight. Such diets put strict estrictions on when, what and how much you can eat. This will lead to eeling constantly hungry and uncomfortable. It is not feasible to maintain hese diets for long, and as soon as you break these diets, you will quickly everse any weight loss, and possibly even gain more weight. A more ractical approach is to have a diet plan that does not leave you hungry, nd one that you can stick to forever. We have many great recipes in the ater section of this book which you can eat plenty of, and keep a part of our diet forever.

Another important measure to maintain healthy metabolism is to et enough sleep and manage your stress. Studies have shown that those vho were consistently sleeping for four hours or less had significantly educed metabolism. Maintaining regular sleep schedule and reducing listractions while falling asleep will help you get good sleep.

Stress is also a negative factor for maintaining a healthy metabolism. For one, stress will adversely affect your sleep. Another reason is that stress releases stress hormones in the body, and constant release of these hormones can cause an increase in belly fat. This is a major risk factor for cardiovascular issues and diabetes. Stress will also increase your appetite causing you to eat more than you need. Sudden weight gain is considered as an indicator of depression.

Some other useful habits for increasing metabolism are consumption of certain beverages such as green tea or black coffee. Note that addition of milk or sugar in these beverages will negate any advantages. Coffee can make you feel more active and thus encourage more physical activity. Research into green tea has shown that it increases your body's metabolism and fat oxidation by small by statistically significant amount.

The antioxidants in coffee and green tea help as well. Another important aspect to remember is to keep hydrated and drink plenty of water. Dehydration will slow down metabolism as a water saving measure by the body. Spicing up your food by hot pepper or chillies will also help you burn more calories. The capsaicin found in many hot spices has a thermogenic effect, that is, it makes your body heat up slightly, burning a few extra calories in the process. You must have breakfast in order to kick start your body's metabolic functions. Having several small meals across the day instead of two large meals is significantly better to maintain a good metabolic rate throughout the day. Avoid alcohol as far as possible. The body burns alcohol before any carbs or sugars, and thus more carbs and sugars may be converted and stored as fats.

Let us have a quick look at the factors that can slow down your metabolism rate.

Hormones

A change in the function or level of your hormones affects your metabolism. For example, thyroid disorder can alter the function of hormones in your body and cause the metabolism to slow down. Stress also disrupts your hormonal function.

Lack of Sleep

Your metabolism rate slows down when you sacrifice your night sleep for the sake of work. It becomes harder for your body to use energy when you keep awake at night.

Eating too less

When you eat too little because you want to lose weight or you are too busy to consume large meals, your body has a fewer supply of calories. Hence, these few calories become the only source of energy to your body and metabolism slows down.

Drinking Less Water

Water keeps your metabolism rate good and when you reduce the intake of water-rich fruits like watermelon and cucumbers or drink less water, your metabolism suffers.

Inadequate Calcium

Your metabolism needs calcium more than your bones. Check your diet when you complain from a slow metabolism and find out if you are taking enough calcium or no.

Drugs

Some drugs which are prescribed for depression or other psychological issues slow down the heartbeat and have other effects which impact metabolism and it also slows down.

Low-Carb Diet

Low-carb diet throughout the time is dangerous because your body does not have enough carb for making insulin. The lack of this important hormone is not a good signal for your metabolism. Hence, it slows down.

Irregular Meals

Mealtimes are important because your body loves you to eat on-time. Changing the time of your meal can play havoc with your metabolism.

Long-Term Stress

During stress hours, your body makes a hormone called cortisol which provides you energy instantly to cope with the stress. So, when you are stressed for long hours, your body keeps making cortisol and automatically avoids making insulin. This is a red light for your metabolism.

Diet Plan for High Metabolism

We shall present a great diet plan which can help you increase your metabolism significantly and lose weight without feeling hungry all the time. The diet plan will include enough food, though overeating will be counterproductive for any weight loss efforts.

Breakfast is your first meal of the day that has a major role in keeping your metabolism rate excellent!

So, go ahead and enjoy unraveling secrets of a new journey to your destination of excellent health and of course, countless benefits like a smart body, healthy skin, strong immunity, more physical strength, better sleep, and above all an enviable long-term sexual ability.

Chapter 1

Breakfast Recipes

We keep our focus on the fact that your metabolism is mainly owed to your breakfast schedule. This first meal of the day keeps your entire day good if you take your breakfast on time and with a good amount of nutrients. Since your metabolism is important for keeping you healthy and fit, you need to find ways to enjoy your breakfast and do not skip it.

Ham Omelette

Prep: 7 Min   Servings: 2   Cook: 5 Min

Eggs - 3

Butter - 3 tbsp

Swiss Cheese - ¼ Cup shredded

Milk - 3 tbsp

Cooked Ham - ½ Cup shredded

Salt and pepper to taste

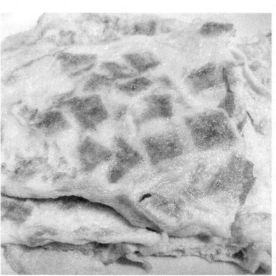

1. Melt the butter in a frying pan.
2. Beat the eggs with milk, salt, and pepper.
3. Spread the mixture in the pan.
4. When the eggs are cooked, spread shredded ham and cheese on the half of omelette and cover it with the other half.
5. Cook for a couple of minutes on medium heat and serve hot.

Nutrition Per Serving:

Calories: 260 kcal	Fat: 8g
Carbs: 2g	Protein: 20g

Peanut Butter Oatmeal

Prep: 0 Min   Servings: 2   Cook: 5
Min

Milk – 1 ½ Cups

Salt - 1 tsp

Old-fashioned Oats - 1 Cup

Creamy Peanut Butter - 2 tbsp

Honey 2 - tbsp

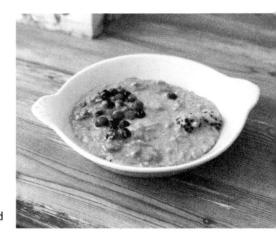

1. In a small saucepan, pour in
   milk to boil and add oats.
2. Cook and stir for five minutes.
3. Once done, turn off the fire and
   add honey and peanut butter.
4. Transfer into a bowl and serve!

Nutrition Per Serving:

Calories: 160 kcal	Fat: 1g
Carbs: 20g	Protein: 6g

Peach & Berries Parfait

Prep: 7 Min   Servings: 4   Cook: 0 Min

Fat-free Vanilla Yogurt - 4 Cups –
½ filled

Medium Peaches - 2 Chopped

Fresh Blackberries - 2 Cups

Granola without raisins - ½ Cup

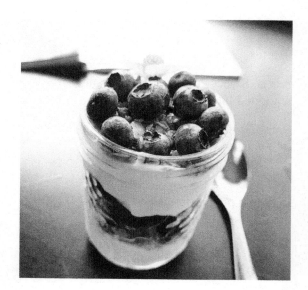

1. Fill all 4 cups with ½ filled
   yogurt.
2. Layer all the ingredients one
   by one in all four cups.
3. Once done, serve and enjoy.

Nutrition Per Serving:

Calories: 60 kcal	Fat: 0g
Carbs: 10g	Protein: 3.5g

Sweet Potato Eggs

Prep: 10 Min   Servings: 2   Cook: 8 Min

Butter - 2 tsp

Large Sweet Potato – 1 boiled and chopped into cubes.

Large Eggs - 4

Goat Cheddar Cheese Shredded - 3 tbsp

Salt and pepper to taste

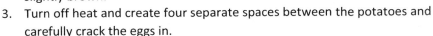

1. Heat a pan and add in butter. Also, preheat oven to 425°F.
2. Add in sweet potatoes and cook for about 4 minutes until slightly brown.
3. Turn off heat and create four separate spaces between the potatoes and carefully crack the eggs in.
4. Sprinkle cheddar cheese and transfer the pan to the oven and bake for 5-7 minutes until the egg begins to set, ensure that the yolk is not overcooked and still runny by lightly shaking the pan.
5. Once done, remove pan from oven and serve with some salt and pepper to as desired.

Nutrition Per Serving:

Calories: 160 kcal	Fat: 9g
Carbs: 4g	Protein: 18g

Cloud Egg

Prep: 5 Min   Servings: 4   Cook: 10 Min

Large Eggs – 4, yolks and whites separated

Italian Seasoning – ¼ tsp

Parmesan Cheese - ¼ Cup shredded

Chives – ¼ cup

Salt and pepper to taste

1. Beat the egg whites with Italian seasoning, salt and pepper until foamy.
2. Grease a skillet and pour the egg mixture in.
3. When half cooked, make 4 ditches in the cooked whites.
4. Sprinkle cheese equally in all four and continue cooking until the cheese is slightly brown.
5. Pour one yolk in each ditch over the cheese and cook for another 3-4 minutes.
6. Once done, sprinkle with chives and serve hot.

Note: Beat the whites very well so that the cooked egg is foamy like clouds.

Nutrition Per Serving:

Calories: 70 kcal	Fat: 0.5g
Carbs: 0g	Protein: 6.5g

Belgian Waffle Eggs

Prep: 7 Min   Servings: 1   Cook: 5 Min

Canadian Bacon - 1 Slice

Large Egg - 1

Spring Onion – 1 Chopped

Belgian Waffles - 2

Reduced-fat shredded cheddar cheese - 1 tbsp

Slices of tomato (optional)

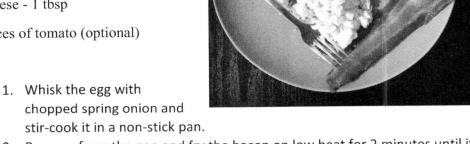

1. Whisk the egg with chopped spring onion and stir-cook it in a non-stick pan.
2. Remove from the pan and fry the bacon on low heat for 2 minutes until it is brown and cooked on both sides.
3. Prepare waffles on a serving plate and place the eggs and bacon along.
4. Serve and enjoy together with the waffles or separately.

Nutrition Per Serving:

Calories: 260 kcal	Fat: 3g
Carbs: 25g	Protein: 18g

Tomato Cups

Prep: 4 Min   Servings: 1   Cook: 15 Min

Large Eggs - 2

Large Plum Tomato – 1, halved
and deseeded

Grated Parmesan cheese - 2 tbsp

Salt and pepper to taste

Mixed Herbs – 2 tbsp, chopped
(optional)

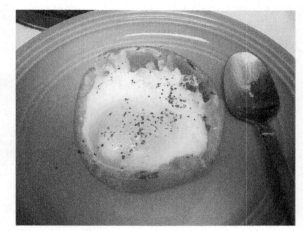

1. Heat oven to 450°F.
2. Place the halved tomatoes on a baking sheet.
3. Crack the eggs and gently place in each of the tomato. Season with salt, pepper and parmesan.
4. Place into the oven and bake for about 6 to 8 minutes until the eggs are set.
5. Once done, serve and enjoy.

Nutrition Per Serving (2 Strips):

Calories: 175 kcal	Fat: 7g
Carbs: 16g	Protein: 9g

Portobello Eggshrooms

Prep: 7 Min   Servings: 4   Cook: 20 Min

Shredded Gouda Cheese – ¼ Cup

Large Portobello Mushrooms - 4, Without stems

Large Eggs - 4

Frozen Creamed Spinach - 2 Packs, 10 oz

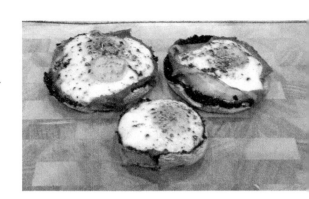

Cooked Crumbled Bacon – ½ Cup

Salt and pepper to taste (optional)

1. Take an ungreased baking pan and place the mushrooms upside down.
2. Divide the spinach on each mushroom with a spoon. Keep it shaped like a bowl.
3. Carefully crack an egg inside the mushroom and sprinkle some cheese on each.
4. Place into the oven and bake for 15 to 20 minutes at 375°. Check frequently so that you can take them out if the eggs are settled early.
5. Once done, sprinkle some bacon, salt and pepper if you like and serve hot!

Nutrition Per Serving:

Calories: 240 kcal	Fat: 3g
Carbs: 10g	Protein: 11g

Chive Omelet with Cream Cheese

Prep: 5 Min   Servings: 2   Cook: 5 Min

Olive oil - 1 tbsp

Large Eggs - 4

Minced Chives - 2 tbsp

Water - 2 tbsp

Cream Cheese - 2 oz.

Salt and pepper to taste

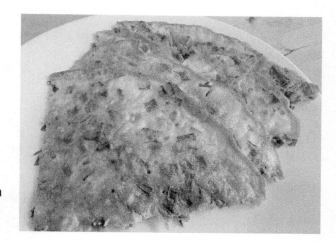

1. Take a large frying pan or a skillet and pour in olive oil to heat over medium heat.
2. Beat the eggs along with chives, salt, pepper, and water.
3. Pour the beaten eggs in the skillet and let the sides set.
4. When the sides are set, push the sides towards the middle, letting the entire omelet cook well.
5. Once done, turn off the heat and sprinkle cream cheese on half of the omelet and fold the other half over the cheese.
6. Slide the omelet on a plate and serve hot.

Nutrition Per Serving:

Calories: 305 kcal	Fat: 25g
Carbs: 2g	Protein: 16g

Banana Pancakes

Prep: 7 Min   Servings: 4   Cook: 6 Min

Whole Wheat Pancake Mix - 2 Cups

Large Banana - 1, mashed

Old-fashioned oats finely chopped – ½ Cup

Chopped Walnuts – ¼ Cup

Milk – ½ Cup

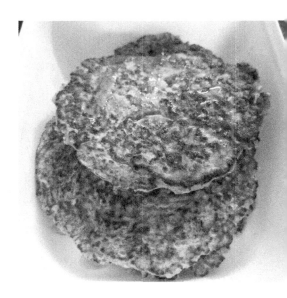

1. Pour the pancake mix in a bowl and beat with milk.
2. Add mashed banana, walnuts, and oats into the mixture.
3. Head the griddle and spray with cooking spray.
4. Pour half-cup of the batter and make four pancakes.
5. When bubbles start appearing, flip over and continue cooking till golden brown.
6. Once done, serve hot.

Nutrition Per Serving:

Calories: 80 kcal	Fat: 2g
Carbs: 13g	Protein: 4g

Granola Fruit Parfait

Prep: 10 Min   Servings: 4   Cook: 0 Min

Reduced-fat, Plain Greek yogurt - 4 Cups

Instant Vanilla **or** Cheesecake Pudding mix - 1 pack

Almond Butter - ½ Cup

Granola with Fruit and Nuts - 1 cup

Fruits (any fruits you prefer)

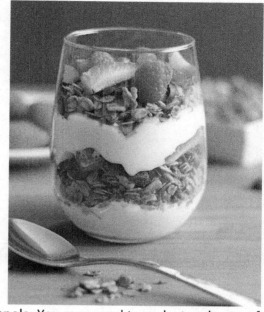

1. Take a large bowl. Add in it yogurt and cheesecake pudding and mix until smooth.
2. Stir in almond butter. Mix well.
3. Take four parfait glasses and layer the yogurt mixture and granola. You may need to make two layers of each.
4. Top with any fruits of your choice. Serve immediately and do not leave for later.

Nutrition Per Serving:

Calories: 500 kcal	Fat: 24g
Carbs: 50g	Protein: 32g

Marmalade French Toast

Prep: 10 Min   Servings: 6   Cook: 7 Min

Whipped Cream Cheese - 1
Container, 8 oz.

Sourdough Bread - 12 Slices

Orange Marmalade – ¾ Cup

Large Eggs - 2

Milk - 2 tbsp

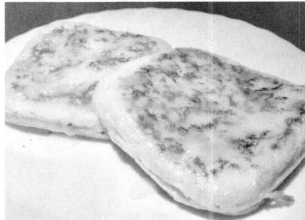

1. Take six slices of bread and layer them with cream cheese.
2. Apply marmalade on the top and take another six slices to cover them in the form of sandwiches.
3. Beat the eggs in a bowl and add milk to it.
4. Take a large flat frying pan or a griddle and slightly grease it. Heat over medium heat.
5. Dip the both sides of the sandwich into the egg mixture and place them on the surface of the griddle or pan.
6. Toast the sandwiches on each side for 2-3 minutes until golden brown.
7. Once done, serve hot and enjoy.

Nutrition Per Serving:

Calories: 440 kcal	Fat: 9g
Carbs: 55g	Protein: 13g

Salami Sandwiches

Prep: 10 Min   Servings: 2   Cook: 10 Min

French Bread - 1 Loaf

Thinly Sliced Hard Salami - 16 Slices

Large Tomato or Lettuce (any vegetables of your choice) - 1, cut into slices

Deli Ham - 8 Slices

Swiss Cheese - 8 Slices

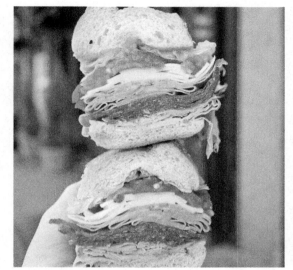

1. Cut the loaf into two equal halves.
2. Now, cut each half into two equal parts.
3. Layer the bottom side of the bread pieces with salami, cheese, ham and vegetables of your choice. Cover them with the top pieces.
4. Toast or bake them on an indoor grill or an oven for 3-4 minutes at 370F or until golden brown. Serve fresh and enjoy.

Nutrition Per Serving:

Calories: 690 kcal	Fat: 29g
Carbs: 55g	Protein: 43g

Eggs and Sausages Wraps

Prep: 10 Min   Servings: 3   Cook: 15 Min

Beef Sausages - 6

Large Eggs - 6

Milk - 2 tbsp

Shredded Cheddar
Cheese - 1 Cup

Flour Tortillas - 6

Toppings: Chopped
Spring Onion,
Cilantro, Green chili
(optional)

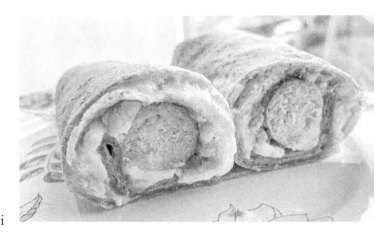

1. Remove the sausages from their casing and cook them over low heat in a greased skillet.
2. In a bowl, whisk the eggs with milk until creamy smooth.
3. Once the sausages are cooked, remove from fire and pour the eggs into the skillet.
4. Cook over low heat until the egg is fully cooked.
5. Add cheese and stir for half a minute and turn off the fire.
6. Divide the mixture for 6 tortillas.
7. Fill each tortilla with eggs and sausages. Add toppings if you like and roll it up; serve them hot.

Nutrition Per Serving:

Calories: 505 kcal	Fat: 30g
Carbs: 28g	Protein: 27g

Instant Cereal Bars

Prep: 10 Min   Servings: 6   Cook: 5 Min

Sugar - 2 Cups

Corn Syrup - 2 Cups

Chunky Peanut Butter - 1 Jar - 40 oz.

Oat Cereal - 6 Cups

Rice Cereal - 6 Cups

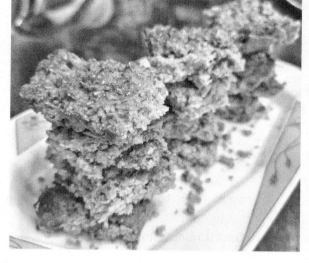

1. Grease two trays lightly and set aside.
2. Take a large pan and boil sugar and corn syrup. Stir constantly till it is fully dissolved and remove from fire.
3. Add in peanut butter and mix well.
4. Stir in both of the cereals and quickly spread onto the greased tray.
5. Level the surface with a spoon as fast as you can and cut into bars while it's hot.
6. Once done, you can serve them at any time. They taste great when they are cold.

Nutrition Per Serving:

Calories: 96 kcal	Fat: 5g
Carbs: 11g	Protein: 4g

Almond Banana Smoothie

Prep: 5 Min   Servings: 2   Cook: 0 Min

Hulled Hemp Seeds – 2 tsp

Natural Almond Butter – 1 ½ tbsp

Frozen Banana – 1, cut into chunks

2% Greek yogurt – ¼ Cup

Unsweetened Vanilla Whey
Protein Powder - 2 tbsp

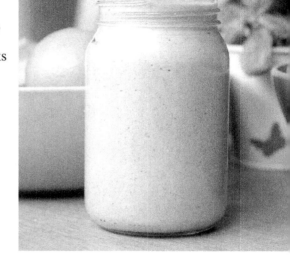

1. In a blender, combine all
   the ingredients and blend
   about 1 minute till frothy.
2. Serve and enjoy.

Nutrition Per Serving:

Calories: 329 kcal	Fat: 1g
Carbs: 24g	Protein: 21g

Scrambled Egg Tortilla

Prep: 5 Min   Servings: 2   Cook: 7 Min

Large Eggs - 4

Corn Tortillas - 4 halved
and cut into strips

Fresh Spinach – ¼ Cup
Chopped

Shredded Reduced-fat
Cheddar Cheese - 2 tbsp

Salt and pepper to taste
(optional)

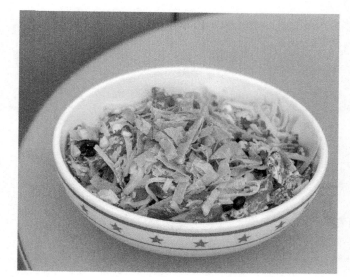

1. Take a large bowl
   and whisk the eggs.
2. Stir in cheese and spinach.
3. Heat a large skillet greased with cooking spray. Keep the heat medium.
4. Pour in the egg mixture and cook while stirring until the eggs are firm.
5. Add in the tortillas and continue cooking while stirring until it turns
   slightly brown.
6. Once done, serve hot and enjoy.

Nutrition Per Serving:

Calories: 150 kcal	Fat: 3g
Carbs: 14g	Protein: 17g

Cinnamon Pancakes

Prep: 7 Min   Servings: 4   Cook: 10 Min

Complete Buttermilk Pancake Mix - 1 Cup

Ground Cinnamon - 1 tsp

Chunky Cinnamon Applesauce - 1 Cup

Butter - 1 Stick

Maple Syrup – ¼ Cup

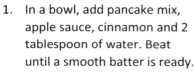

1. In a bowl, add pancake mix, apple sauce, cinnamon and 2 tablespoon of water. Beat until a smooth batter is ready.
2. Heat a griddle and grease it with butter.
3. Pour in ¼ of the batter and make four pancakes.
4. Flip them when bubbles arise and cook both sides till it turns brown.
5. Remove and place the pancakes in a plate. Pour in maple syrup and serve.

Nutrition Per Serving:

Calories: 70 kcal	Fat: 1g
Carbs: 15g	Protein: 2g

Fruit Yogurt

Prep: 7 Min   Servings: 4   Cook: 0 Min

Cut-up Fresh Fruit (strawberries, raspberry, blueberry, dates, etc) 4 – ½ Cups

Vanilla or Lemon yogurt - 2 Cups

Honey - 1 tbsp

Grated Orange Zest – ½ tsp

Almond Extract – ¼ tsp

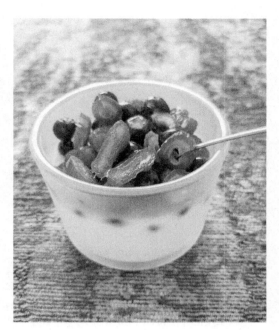

1. Set the fruit pieces in 4 equal serving glass bowls or cups.
2. Mix the yogurt with orange zest and honey.
3. Spoon the yogurt mixture over the fruits and serve.

Nutrition Per Serving:

Calories: 95 kcal	Fat: 0g
Carbs: 20g	Protein: 2g

Chicken Oatmeal Porridge

Prep: 10 Min   Servings: 2   Cook: 20 Min

Boneless Chicken Breast - 2, cut into pieces

Rolled Oats – 1 Cup

Butter – 1 tbsp

Crushed Garlic – 1 tbsp

Bay Leaves – 3

Salt and pepper to taste

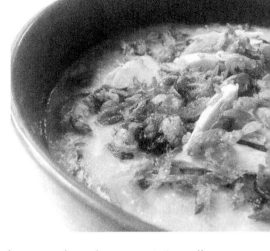

1. In a non-stick pan, heat oil and add garlic, bay leaves and sauté for a minute.
2. Add in chicken pieces, oats and some salt and pepper. Mix well.
3. Add 2 cups of water and stir evenly.
4. Cook until the chicken is done.
5. Add in butter and mix well.
6. Once done, transfer the porridge into a serving bowl and garnish with any toppings you desire and enjoy.

Nutrition Per Serving:

Calories: 150 kcal	Fat: 2g
Carbs: 15g	Protein: 24g

Fresh Omelette

Prep: 10 Min   Servings: 5   Cook: 20 Min

Large Eggs - 10

Butter - 6 tbsp

Fresh or Frozen Corn, thawed - 1 Cup

Shredded Cheddar Cheese – ½ Cup

Fresh Tomatoes Diced – ½ Cup (Optional)

Salt and pepper to taste

1. In a large bowl, whisk eggs, salt and pepper.
2. Heat a large non-stick skillet and add 4 tbsp butter.
3. Add corn and cook till tender.
4. Remove the corn from the pan and add 2 tbsp of butter. Keep the heat medium-high.
5. Pour in half of the beaten eggs. Push the edges inside and let the eggs cook evenly.
6. When the eggs are set, sprinkle half of the shredded cheddar cheese and corn on half of the omelette and fold the other half over the cheese.
7. Cook for a couple of minutes and transfer the omelette onto a plate.
8. Repeat the same with the rest of the eggs, corn and cheese. Serve hot with diced tomatoes if you like.

Nutrition Per Serving:

Calories: 203 kcal	Fat: 23g
Carbs: 5g	Protein: 20g

Fruit Toasts

Prep: 10 Min   Servings: 1   Cook: 0 Min

Non-fat Strawberry Greek yogurt - 4 tbsp

Cream Cheese - 2 tbsp

100% Whole-wheat Bread - 2 Slices, toasted

Fruits - 1, strawberry, blueberry, avocado (any fruits of your choice)

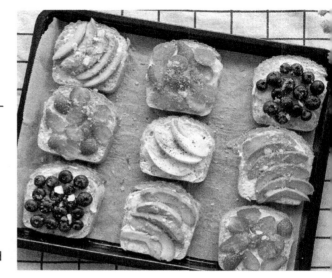

1. Beat the yogurt and cream cheese.
   Spread them on the toasted bread.
2. Arrange pieces of strawberry, blueberry, avocado, or any fruit of your choice equally on both slices.
3. Serve with cold milk or orange juice if you like!

Nutrition Per Serving:

Calories: 185 kcal	Fat: 1g
Carbs: 23g	Protein: 9g

Corn Tortillas

Prep: 7 Min   Servings: 2   Cook: 5 Min

Corn Tortillas - 2

Eggs - 2

Salsa - 1 tbsp

Shredded Cheddar
Cheese - 2 tbsp

Salt and pepper to
taste

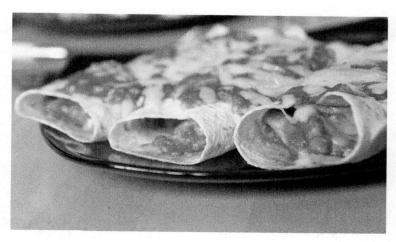

1. Spread the tortillas with salsa and cheese.
2. Heat them in the microwave and remove when the cheese is melted, around 30 seconds.
3. Meanwhile, heat up a skillet and spray it with cooking spray.
4. Pour in eggs and cook over medium heat, keep stirring.
5. When the eggs are cooked, spread them on the tortillas and serve.

Nutrition Per Serving:

Calories: 115 kcal	Fat: 3.5g
Carbs: 12g	Protein: 11g

Hazelnut Chocolate Sandwiches

Prep: 5 Min   Servings: 4   Cook: 15 Min

Large Eggs - 4

Whole Milk - 1 Cup

Wholewheat Bread - 8 slices

Chocolate Hazelnut Spread - 8
tbsp

Butter - 3 tbsp

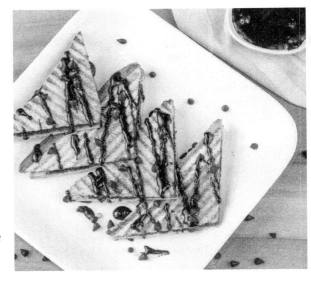

1. In a bowl, whisk the eggs with milk. Set aside and heat some butter in a skillet.
2. Dip the slices one by one in the eggs and place them on a heated skillet.
3. Golden brown the slices on both sides and place them on a plate.
4. Apply 1 tbsp of chocolate-hazelnut spread on each slice and make one sandwich.
5. Repeat the same with other slices. Serve hot.

Nutrition Per Serving:

Calories: 167 kcal	Fat: 6g
Carbs: 22g	Protein: 19g

Skinny Sausage Patty

Prep: 10 Min   Servings: 8   Cook:
0 Min

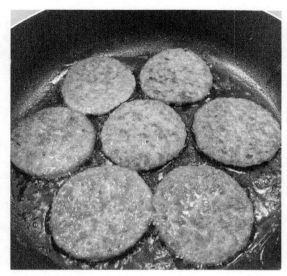

Lean Ground Turkey or Chicken –
 lb (cage-free)

Ground Black Pepper – ½ tsp

Garlic Powder – ½ tsp

Dried Oregano – 1 tsp

Crushed Red Pepper Flakes - 1 tsp
(optional)

Sea Salt to taste (optional)

1. Mix all the ingredients in a large bowl.
2. Make about 8 patties and heat up a non-stick skillet on medium heat.
3. Place the patties on the skillet and cooked until brown on both sides and cooked through.
4. Once done, serve on a plate and enjoy with desired toppings.

Nutrition Per Serving:

Calories: 82 kcal	Fat: 3g
Carbs: 0g	Protein: 11g

Fruity Quinoa

Prep: 10 Min   Servings: 4   Cook: 15 Min

Almond Milk - 4 Cups

Quinoa - 1 Cup mixed (equal parts of white, red, and black varieties)

Fresh Strawberries or Blueberries - 10 oz (you can choose your choice of fruit)

Pistachios - 2 tbsp, sliced (you can replace with any other nut of your choice)

Honey - 1 tbsp

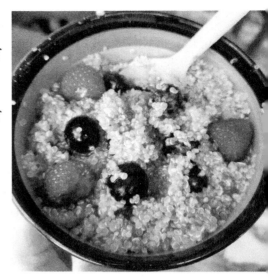

1. Boil quinoa until fully soft.
2. Pour it into a bowl and add in almond milk and honey, Mix well.
3. Garnish with any fruit and nuts of your choice.
4. Serve immediately or later.

Nutrition Per Serving:

Calories: 130 kcal	Fat: 0.5g
Carbs: 4g	Protein: 7g

Chorizo and Sweet Potato Hash

Prep: 20 Min   Servings: 4   Cook: 30 Min

Olive oil - 2 tbsp

Fully Cooked Spanish Chorizo, ½ lb finely chopped

Finely Chopped Sweet Potatoes - 4 Cups (about 2 medium)

Finely Chopped Onion - 1 Medium

Finely Chopped Minced Garlic - 4 Cloves

Salt and pepper to taste

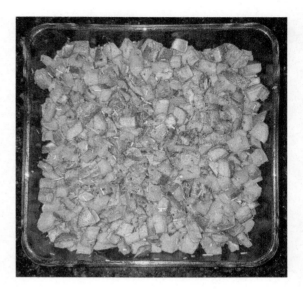

1. Put your Dutch oven over medium-high heat.
2. Add olive oil and chorizo. Cook and keep stirring until golden brown and add in the remaining ingredients.
3. Reduce heat to medium-low and continue cooking for 20 minutes but do not cover.
4. Once the sweet potatoes are soft and cooked, pour into bowls of 4 and serve hot!

Nutrition Per Serving:

Calories: 205 kcal	Fat: 1g
Carbs: 15g	Protein: 9g

Green Tea Fruit Smoothie

Prep: 4 Min   Servings: 1   Cook: 0 Min

Frozen Banana – 1

Frozen Strawberries – 4

Frozen Kiwi – 1, peeled

Kale – 2 Cups (organic)

Green Tea – 1 ½ Cup (No sweeteners added)

Ice Cubes - 5

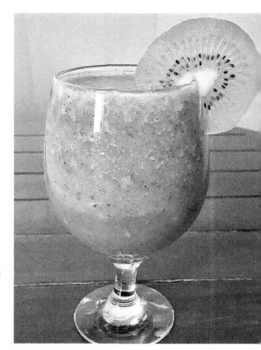

1. Combine all ingredients into a blender and blend for 1 minute or until smooth.
2. Once done, serve and enjoy.

Nutrition Per Serving:

Calories: 185 kcal	Fat: 1g
Carbs: 40g	Protein: 7g

Overnight Fruit Oats

Prep: 5 Min
Min

Servings: 1

Cook: 0

Oats - 1/3 Cup (gluten-free or regular)

Almond Milk – ½ Cup

Chia Seeds - 1 tsp

Maple Syrup – ½ tsp

Mix fruit of your choice, 1 Cup, sliced

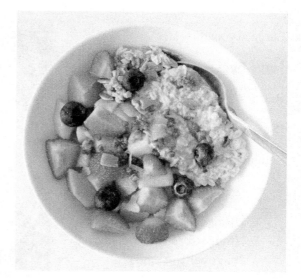

1. In an airtight container, mix chia seeds, oats, almond milk, and maple syrup.
2. Closed the lid tightly and place the container in the fridge overnight.
3. In the morning, pour the oats into a bowl and stir well.
4. Top with sliced fruits. Serve cool!

Nutrition Per Serving:

Calories: 270 kcal	Fat: 0g
Carbs: 47g	Protein: 5g

Avocado Egg Breakfast

Prep: 10 Min   Servings: 2   Cook: 10 Min

Large Avocado - 1

Large Eggs - 2

Butter - 2 tbsp

Bread - 4 Slices

Salt and pepper to taste

1. Bring a pot of water to boil (make sure water is enough to cover the eggs).
2. Place metal rims (outer rim) of two mason jars lids into the pot and lay flat.
3. Crack the eggs into a separate bowl.
4. Once the water boils, turn off the heat and place the bowls into the pot of water. Cover the pot and poach for about 5 minutes.
5. Meanwhile, toast the bread and spread half of the avocado on each slice.
6. Once the eggs are done, place them onto the toast and sprinkle with salt and pepper. Serve and enjoy.

Nutrition Per Serving:

Calories: 120 kcal	Fat: 5g
Carbs: 25g	Protein: 10g

BONUS

i, my dear readers. Thank you so much for your continuous support as it
ally meant a lot to me. In case you have missed out "Quick & Easy
letabolism Miracle Diet: Shed Stubborn Fats with 5 Ingredient or Less"
3ook 1), I will be sharing some of the recipes and information which is
adily available in the book with just a click away. Thank you once again.

Breakfast Recipes

Buckwheat pancake

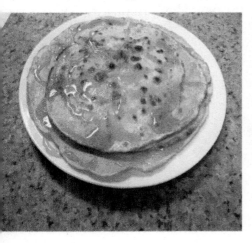

Buckwheat is a cereal and hence it
is rich in carbohydrates, and it is
also rich in fibre. A unique
advantage of buckwheat is that it is
gluten-free, making it ideal for
people with celiac disease. This also
makes use of some eggs and milk,
thus adding some proteins.

ervings: 4

gredients

ıckwheat flour – 1 cup

ɡg white, beaten – 1

ce milk – 1 cup

ɑking powder – 2 tsp

ɔices and seasoning – cinnamon powder, vanilla extract, sweetener (optional,
ɔu can use sugar or artificial sweetener)

1. Mix all the dry ingredients in a large mixing bowl.
2. Take another bowl and beat the egg whites in it, then add the milk, some oil and vanilla extract to it and mix well.
3. Add the dry ingredient mix to this and mix it well into a smooth batter.
4. Grease a non-stick griddle or a skillet over medium heat.
5. Use about ¼ cups of batter per pancake. Cook it until you see bubbles on top and then flip it.
6. Cook both sides until brown. Your pancakes are now ready to serve.

Nutrition Per Serving:

Calories: 51 kcal	Fat: 1.4g
Carbs: 6.5g	Protein: 2.3g

Pineapple and Coconut Smoothie

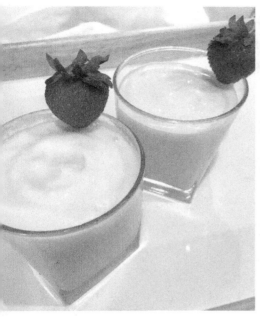

This is a delicious smoothie which blends pineapple with coconut. There are a few carbs in this smoothie, so it must not be consumed frequently. But the abundance of proteins makes this suitable for the high protein phase. Chia seeds, in addition to Greek yoghurt, make this an excellent protein-rich shake.

Servings: 4

Ingredients

Buckwheat flour – 1 cup

Egg white, beaten – 1

Rice milk – 1 cup

Baking powder – 2 tsp

Spices and seasoning – cinnamon powder, vanilla extract, sweetener (optional, you can use sugar or artificial sweetener)

1. Soak the chia seeds in water for 8 hours before preparation so that they expand and become soft. You can leave them overnight in a covered container in a refrigerator.
2. For smoothie preparation, toss all the ingredients into a blender and blend to the desired texture. Save the coconut flakes for the last to add some nice texture.
3. If you like your smoothie cold, use frozen pineapple chunks or add some ice cubes and blend.

Nutrition Per Serving:

Calories: 51 kcal	Fat: 1.4g
Carbs: 6.5g	Protein: 2.3g

Steak and Asparagus Lettuce Wraps

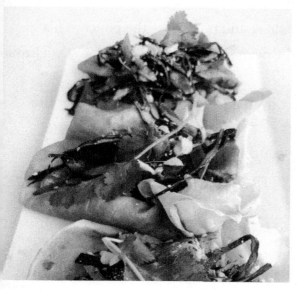

This is a delicious recipe that will be a great meal. Asparagus is good for filling the stomach without too many calories. It has healthy fibre though. Lettuce is rich in minerals and vitamins, especially Vitamin A. The steak will ensure that there are enough proteins in the meal.

Servings: 2

Ingredients

Asparagus – 8 spears

Round steak, cut into strips – 280 to 300 gm, or about 10 oz

Romaine – 4 leaves

Spices and seasonings – minced garlic, lime juice, dried cilantro, red pepper flakes, mustard or balsamic vinegar, salt and pepper

1. Prepare the oven and the broiler pan by preheating it.

2. Make a pouch for the steak and asparagus. You can use foil for making the pouch. In a mixing bowl, mix the lime juice, minced garlic, red pepper flakes, dried cilantro, salt and pepper to make spice liquid.

3. Drizzle this liquid over the steak and then close the pouch. This pouch must be broiled in the oven for 25 minutes. Let the steak broil longer if it is not done.

4. Remove the pouch from the oven and open one end to let out the steam.

5. Empty the contents of this pouch in a bowl. You can add more of that spice liquid or add other spices like mustard, or a bit of vinegar, as per your taste.

6. Take the romaine leaves and lay them down on a plate. Put the mixture on top of it, and cover with another romaine leaf.

7. Roll it up to make a wrap, and it is ready to serve.

Nutrition Per Serving:

Calories: 206 kcal	Fat: 5.7g
Carbs: 4g	Protein: 34g

Roasted Chicken

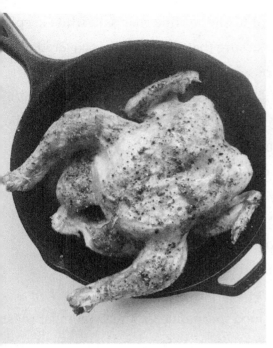

This is plain and simple salted and roasted chicken. It can be prepared just with chicken and salt for seasoning. Having just chicken as a meal will ensure that you get plenty of proteins.

Servings: 4

Ingredients

Chicken – 1 whole, 1.5 to 1.8 kg or about 3.5 to 4 lbs

Kosher or fine rock salt – as required

1. Wash the chicken and then dry it, make sure that the chicken is completely dry, use paper towels to dry it.
2. Sprinkle generous quantity of Kosher or fine rock salt, while keeping your hand away from it. Make sure that the chicken is covered with salt completely, from both outside and inside.
3. Take a wire rack and place it on a baking tray. Place the chicken on the tray and chill it in the refrigerator overnight. This will allow the seasoning to be absorbed in the chicken.
4. Take it out of the refrigerator and let it sit outside for an hour to reach room temperature. Meanwhile, preheat your oven to 425° F.
5. Put the chicken in the oven to roast it. If you have a food thermometer handy, then measure the temperature inside the thickest part of the chicken.
6. Roast it till the temperature at this part reaches about 165° F or higher. If you do not have a food thermometer, then you must roast the chicken for at least 40-50 minutes. You can try to get an idea whether it is cooked or not by piercing it with a fork.
7. Remove the chicken from the oven and let it sit for at least 15 minutes. You can now carve and serve the chicken.

Nutrition Per Serving:

Calories: 503 kcal	Fat: 32g

Spinach Zucchini Ravioli

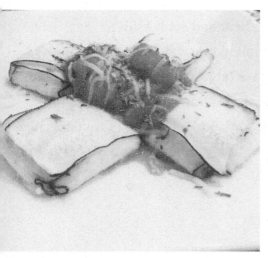

This dish is based on ground turkey as its main ingredient, and thus has plenty of proteins. Spinach adds a lot of micronutrients such as iron, various other minerals and vitamins as well as dietary fibre. Zucchini also has various essential micronutrients.

Servings: 4

Ingredients

Ground turkey – 700 gm or about 1.5 lb

Fresh spinach, chopped – 2 cups

Onion, chopped – 1 small or ½ cup

Zucchini – cut into thin strips, 4 required pre-ravioli

Spices and seasoning – tomato sauce, olive oil, chopped garlic, salt and pepper as desired

1. Sauté the chopped onion, ground turkey, chopped spinach, 1-2 cloves of chopped garlic and other seasonings such as salt and pepper.
2. Mix well and sauté till the turkey is completely cooked. Once the mixture is cooked, turn off the heat and set it aside.
3. Lay down the 2 slices of zucchini in one way and 2 slices across, forming a sort of a cross. Lay 1-2 tablespoon of the cooked mixture in the middle of the cross and them wrap it to form a ravioli.
4. Place it face down in a baking tray. Add a topping of tomato sauce and then set it to bake at 350° F for 30 minutes and it's ready to be served.

Nutrition Per Serving:

Calories: 194 kcal	Fat: 10g
Carbs: 4g	Protein: 21g

Turkey Patty

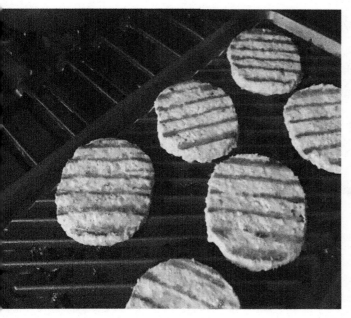

The burger is a classic and a very versatile dish. We shall replace the usual ingredients with healthier ones for making patty for use in burgers. The ground turkey and egg whites will provide plenty of proteins. When consumed with multigrain burger buns as a hamburger, it also provides a good amount of carbs and fibre.

Servings: 4

Ingredients

Ground turkey – 450 gm or about 1 lb

Egg white – 1 egg

Parsley, chopped – ¼ cup

Onion, chopped – ¼ cup

1. Take a large bowl and mix the ground turkey, chopped onion, minced garlic, egg white, parsley, salt and pepper.
2. Take 6 portions from this mixture and shape them into patties with your hand.
3. Cook the patties until done on a grill or a skillet on medium heat with coconut oil and you're ready to serve.

Nutrition Per Serving:

Calories: 251 kcal	Fat: 14.4g
Carbs: 6.2g	Protein: 22.9g

Kiwi Lime Sorbet

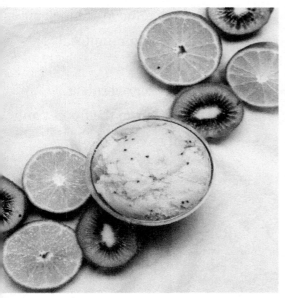

This delicious Kiwi Lime Sorbet will be sure to delight you during a hot summer day. Kiwi will provide you with some carbohydrates and plenty of dietary fibres.

Servings: 4

Ingredients

Kiwis – 10

Lime juice – ¼ cup

Xylitol – ¾ cup

1. Cut all the kiwis into half and remove the kiwi flesh. You can do this by using a spoon roughly the size of the kiwis to scoop the flesh out.
2. Put all the kiwi flesh into a blender and give it a few bursts of spin.
3. Add the Xylitol, lime juice and give it a short spin.
4. Pour the blended mixture into a freezer bag, remove as much air as possible and put it in the freezer for about 45-50 minutes.
5. Remove it and churn it in an ice-cream machine.
6. Scoop it out and freeze the scoops in the freezer overnight. Or at least 5-6 hours. After that, you can remove it from the freezer and serve.

Nutrition Per Serving:

Calories: 124 kcal	Fat: 1g
Carbs: 60g	Protein: 2g

Kale Crisps

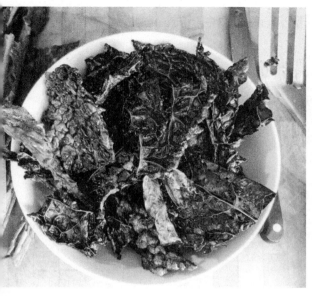

This is a nice snack to munch on when you feel the urge to do so. Kale has very few carbohydrates, an amount of protein and plenty of vitamins.

Servings: 6

Ingredients

Kale – 1 bunch

Spices and seasonings – chilli powder, pepper, sea salt, ground ginger

1. Preheat the oven to 225° F. Loosen up the bunch of kale and tear it into large pieces.
2. Lay down the pieces on a non-stick cooking paper on a baking tray. Season with chilli powder, sea salt, pepper and ground ginger as necessary.
3. Bake it for 8-10 minutes till the colour of the kale turns to darker green and it turns crispy. Kale crisps can now be served.

Nutrition Per Serving:

Calories: 10 kcal	Fat: 0.5g
Carbs: 1.3g	Protein: 0.5g

Check Out Other Books

Quick & Easy Metabolism Miracle Diet:
Shed Stubborn Fats With 5 Ingredients or Less (BOOK 1)

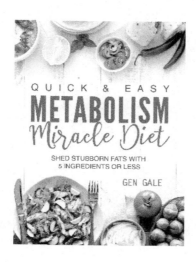

Best Seller: https://www.amazon.com/dp/B074CDRFLS

The 5-Ingredient Keto Fat Bombs Cookbook:
Lose Up to 20 Pounds with 20-Minute Mouthwatering Recipes

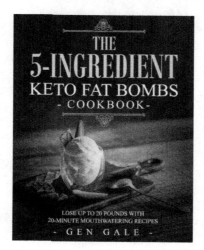

https://www.amazon.com/dp/B07RS4FR9J

5-Ingredient Ketogenic Air Fryer Cookbook for Dummies:
30-Minute Quick, Healthy & Easy Mouthwatering Low-Carb Recipes

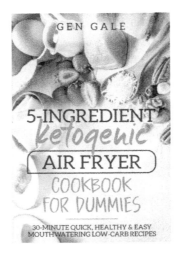

https://www.amazon.com/dp/B07MM65Z2L

5-Ingredient Ketogenic Diet Cookbook with 30-Minute Recipes:
Mouthwatering Low-Carb Recipes for Busy People

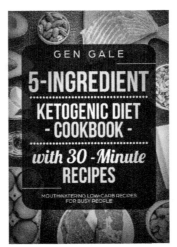

https://www.amazon.com/dp/B07DMWWTF7

The Ultimate Ketogenic Lifestyle:
14 Day Fat Burning, Delicious Low Carb Recipes For Breakfast, Lunch & Dinner

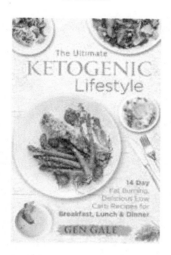

https://www.amazon.com/dp/B01MR01ELG

The 5 Ingredient or Less Ketogenic Instant Pot Cookbook:
Get Lean & Healthy With Mouthwatering
Breakfast, Lunch, Dinner, Soup & Dessert Recipes

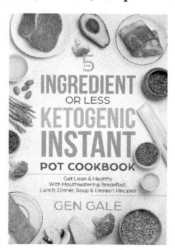

https://www.amazon.com/dp/B079Z3LTJX

What Makes Us Fat:
Change Your Lifestyle In 7 Days

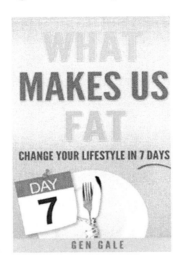

https://www.amazon.com/dp/B01N3UWOYX

Printed in Great Britain
by Amazon

22466032R00040